COMPLETE FORMULA FOR INTERMITTENT FASTING

The Ultimate Weight Loss Diet Guide To Heal Your Body

Giant Success

Copyright © 2023

This publication is protected by copyright law, and no part of it can be reproduced, distributed, or transmitted without written permission, except for brief quotations in reviews and certain noncommercial uses permitted by copyright law. The information provided is for educational purposes only and should not be seen as a substitute for professional medical advice.

The author's views are not necessarily endorsed by others mentioned, and references to products or services are for informational purposes only. Efforts have been made to respect copyright laws and attribute sources properly. The author and publisher are not responsible for any loss or damage resulting from the use of this information. Unauthorized use is strictly prohibited. Thank you for respecting intellectual property rights.

Table of content

INTRODUCTION

Why is Intermittent Fasting Gaining Tremendous Popularity?

The issue of obesity is on the rise, prompting a growing number of individuals to seek effective weight loss methods. Traditional calorie-restricted diets often prove futile for many people due to the difficulty of long-term adherence.

Consequently, this leads to a frustrating cycle of weight loss and regain, commonly known as yo-yo dieting. Apart from potential mental health repercussions, this pattern often results in additional weight gain.

Given these circumstances, it's unsurprising that numerous individuals have been actively exploring a sustainable dietary approach. Enter intermittent fasting, a distinctive lifestyle change rather than a conventional eating plan.

Many adherents of intermittent fasting find it remarkably manageable for extended periods, and, even more impressively, it facilitates effective weight loss.

However, the merits of this eating regimen extend beyond weight management. Many proponents of intermittent fasting believe it offers a range of other health and wellness benefits.

Some enthusiasts even claim that it enhances productivity and focus, enabling them to achieve greater success in their professional lives. Media outlets have recently featured stories about CEOs attributing their accomplishments to intermittent fasting.

Yet, the advantages of intermittent fasting go even further. There is some evidence suggesting that it positively influences blood sugar levels and boosts immunity. Additionally, it may enhance brain function, reduce inflammation, and promote cellular repair within the body.

Considering these compelling factors, it's no wonder that the popularity of intermittent fasting as a dietary approach is on the rise. In the following sections, we will delve deeper into the mechanisms behind intermittent fasting's effectiveness in promoting weight loss.

We will explore the extensive range of benefits offered by this lifestyle change, along with providing guidance on how to embark on this diet protocol.

CHAPTER 1

Understanding Intermittent Fasting

Intermittent fasting is quickly gaining popularity among individuals aiming to shed excess weight. However, it is also embraced by many others seeking to enjoy its numerous health and wellness advantages. So, what exactly is intermittent fasting?

How is Intermittent Fasting Distinct from Other Dietary Approaches?

Intermittent fasting (IF) is essentially a eating pattern rather than a conventional diet. Unlike standard diets that focus on specific foods or calorie restrictions, IF revolves around when you eat.

Traditional diets often lead individuals to obsess over what they can or cannot consume, forbidding fatty and sugary foods and placing heavy emphasis on vegetables, fruits, and low-fat, low-sugar meals.

Those who follow such diets often find themselves daydreaming about indulgent treats and snacks, and although they may lose weight, sticking to the plan in the long run becomes challenging.

Intermittent fasting takes a different approach. It is a lifestyle rather than a strict diet regimen. It involves cycling between periods of fasting and eating, without being fixated on the specific foods being consumed.

This freedom allows individuals to enjoy their favorite foods without guilt. Many people also find that intermittent fasting fits more seamlessly into their lifestyles. However, it is important to be aware of potential challenges when using IF as a weight loss method.

The Origins of Intermittent Fasting

While intermittent fasting as a lifestyle choice is relatively modern, the practice of fasting itself has a long history. Religious texts such as the Bible and the Quran contain references to fasting for spiritual reasons, and many religious individuals continue to fast to this day. The month of Ramadan, during which Muslims abstain from eating from sunrise to sunset, exemplifies the influence of fasting in religious contexts.

Fasting was also practiced in ancient Greek civilizations and held significance in various primitive cultures as part of rituals. Additionally, fasting served as a means of political protest, as exemplified by the suffragettes during the early 20th century.

Therapeutic fasting gained popularity in the 1800s as a preventive and curative measure for various health conditions. Under medical supervision, tailored fasting regimens were utilized to treat ailments ranging from hypertension to headaches.

These fasts could range from a single day to as long as three months.

Although fasting lost popularity with the development of new medications, it has recently experienced a resurgence. In 2019, "intermittent fasting" was among the most commonly searched terms. So, what should you know about it?

The Most Popular Types of Intermittent Fasting

Numerous types of intermittent fasting have gained popularity, each with its dedicated followers. However, they all share the fundamental principle of restricting food intake for a specific period. The duration of the fasting period and the gap between eating windows vary.

One of the most popular IF methods is the 16:8 fast, which involves an eight-hour eating window followed by a 16-hour fasting period. Many individuals find this method convenient as they can easily fit it into their lifestyle by skipping either breakfast or dinner.

Another well-known IF option is the 24-hour fast, also referred to as the Eat-Stop-Eat method. It entails eating normally for one day and then abstaining from food for the subsequent 24 hours. The duration between fasts can range from as short as 24 hours to as long as 72 hours.

The 5:2 fasting method is also favored by many. It involves eating normally for five days of the week, while restricting calorie intake to around 500-600 calories on the other two consecutive days.

Some individuals choose the 20:4 method, wherein they concentrate all their daily eating within a four-hour window, while abstaining from calories for the remaining 20 hours of the day.

There are several other fasting variations, including extended fasts lasting up to 48 or 36 hours, and even longer periods of fasting. If you are considering trying intermittent fasting, it is crucial to select the method that suits you best.

Why is Intermittent Fasting Preferred?

Unlike many other dieting approaches, intermittent fasting allows individuals to enjoy a wide variety of foods without strict limitations. They can indulge in sugary or fatty foods without worry and dine out without counting calories.

They are not compelled to consume foods they dislike or feel deprived of the things they love. It is easy to understand why intermittent fasting has become a popular choice.

Moreover, intermittent fasting offers a multitude of benefits beyond weight loss. It enhances focus and productivity, promotes a sense of well-being, and boosts energy levels.

With these overall wellness advantages, it is no surprise that people prefer intermittent fasting over conventional diets.

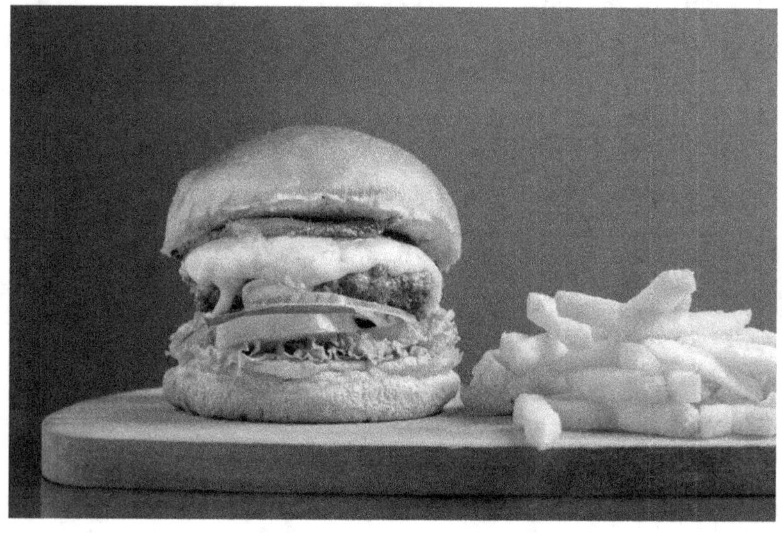

CHAPTER 2

Unveiling the Advantages of Intermittent Fasting

The followers of intermittent fasting have reported numerous benefits associated with this lifestyle. Let's delve deeper into some of the most prevalent advantages.

Weight Loss

Many individuals embrace intermittent fasting as a means to achieve rapid weight loss. Evidence suggests that this eating pattern can indeed expedite the shedding of pounds. Several mechanisms contribute to the weight loss benefits of intermittent fasting.

Firstly, it enhances metabolic function, leading to accelerated fat burning. Moreover, it reduces overall calorie intake by regulating hormones such as insulin, growth hormone, and norepinephrine, which promote fat breakdown and utilization for energy.

Short-term fasting has been found to increase metabolic rate by up to 14 percent, resulting in a higher calorie expenditure. As a result, intermittent fasting can lead to weight loss of up to 8 percent over a period of 3 to 24 weeks—an impressive achievement.

Additionally, individuals who practice intermittent fasting experience a significant reduction in waist circumference, indicating a reduction in harmful belly fat. Notably, intermittent fasting also helps preserve muscle mass compared to calorie restriction diets, which can contribute to a more favorable body composition.

Cellular Repair

During fasting periods, the body initiates a process known as autophagy, wherein cells eliminate waste and metabolize dysfunctional proteins that have accumulated over time.

This cellular cleansing mechanism holds profound benefits, as experts believe it provides protection against various diseases, including Alzheimer's and cancer.

By adopting an intermittent fasting regimen, individuals may enhance their cellular health and potentially extend their lifespan while enjoying improved overall well-being.

Improved Insulin Sensitivity

The prevalence of type 2 diabetes is escalating due to the rising rates of obesity. Insulin resistance, characterized by elevated blood sugar levels, lies at the core of this metabolic disorder.

Intermittent fasting has been shown to significantly improve insulin sensitivity, thereby reducing blood sugar levels. Studies involving human participants have demonstrated a decrease in blood sugar levels of up to 6 percent during fasting periods.

Additionally, fasting insulin levels can drop by as much as 31 percent, lowering the risk of developing type 2 diabetes. Furthermore, research conducted on diabetic laboratory animals indicates that intermittent fasting offers protective effects against kidney damage, a severe complication associated with diabetes.

Therefore, intermittent fasting holds promise as a valuable approach for individuals with diabetes.

Enhanced Brain Function

What benefits the body often benefits the brain as well. Intermittent fasting is known to improve various metabolic factors crucial for optimal brain health.

It reduces oxidative stress, inflammation, and blood sugar levels while enhancing insulin sensitivity, all of which contribute to improved cognitive function. Studies conducted on laboratory rats have also demonstrated that intermittent fasting stimulates the growth of new nerve cells and increases the levels of brain-derived neurotrophic factor (BDNF)—a crucial brain hormone.

Insufficient BDNF levels have been linked to brain disorders and depression. By practicing intermittent fasting, individuals can enhance their brain protection and potentially mitigate these issues.

Furthermore, animal studies have revealed that intermittent fasting can safeguard the brain against damage caused by strokes. These findings collectively indicate that intermittent fasting offers significant benefits for brain health.

Reduced Inflammation

Oxidative stress, characterized by the damaging effects of unstable molecules called free radicals on important molecules like DNA and proteins, plays a key role in chronic diseases and aging. Intermittent fasting has been shown in several studies to enhance the body's resilience against oxidative stress and combat inflammation, which is a driving force behind numerous common diseases.

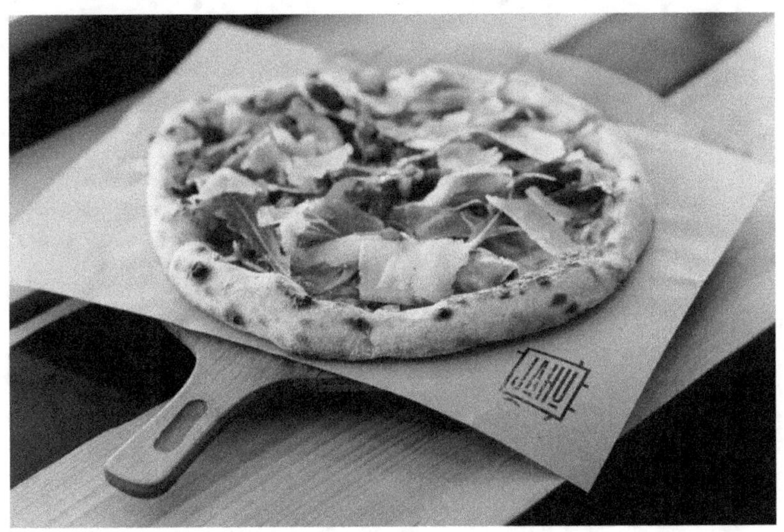

CHAPTER 3

The Mechanisms Behind Intermittent Fasting's Weight Loss Benefits

Weight loss is one of the primary goals of intermittent fasting, and there are three main reasons why this eating pattern promotes effective weight loss.

Reduced Calorie Intake

The key factor contributing to weight loss during intermittent fasting is the reduction in overall calorie intake. With a limited eating window, individuals naturally have less time to consume meals. Typically, one or more meals are skipped each day to adhere to the fasting schedule.

As a result, the total number of calories consumed within a 24-hour period decreases. Creating a calorie deficit is essential for weight loss, and intermittent fasting helps achieve this deficit more effectively.

It is worth noting that some individuals may not experience weight loss with intermittent fasting if they fail to reduce their calorie intake during their eating window. If they continue to eat as much as they would normally, the necessary calorie deficit for weight loss is not achieved.

To ensure weight loss, it is crucial to avoid excessive eating during the eating window and maintain a calorie deficit.

Hormonal Changes that Boost Metabolism

During fasting, the body undergoes various hormonal and metabolic changes to make stored energy more accessible. These changes involve the activity of the nervous system and significant alterations in key hormones.

The following metabolic changes occur during fasting:

Insulin: Insulin levels increase when you eat, but fasting leads to a significant decrease in insulin levels. Lower insulin levels facilitate fat burning.

Human Growth Hormone (HGH): Fasting triggers a substantial increase in HGH levels, potentially reaching up to five times its normal level. HGH promotes muscle gain and fat loss.

Noradrenaline (Norepinephrine): The nervous system sends noradrenaline to fat cells during fasting, stimulating the breakdown of body fat into free fatty acids. These fatty acids are then utilized as a source of energy.

Contrary to the misconception that fasting slows down metabolism, evidence suggests that short-term fasting can actually increase fat burning. Studies have shown that fasting for 48 hours can boost metabolism by up to 14 percent.

Reduced Insulin Levels Accelerate Fat Burning

Insulin, a hormone produced by the pancreas, plays a vital role in converting sugar (glucose) in the bloodstream into energy for cellular fuel. Additionally, insulin promotes the storage of fat in the body.

Whenever you eat, insulin levels rise, but fasting leads to a decrease in insulin levels. Lower insulin levels help prevent excessive fat storage and facilitate the mobilization of stored fat for energy utilization. This can accelerate fat loss and contribute to more rapid weight loss.

By understanding the mechanisms behind intermittent fasting's weight loss benefits, individuals can optimize their approach and maximize their weight loss potential.

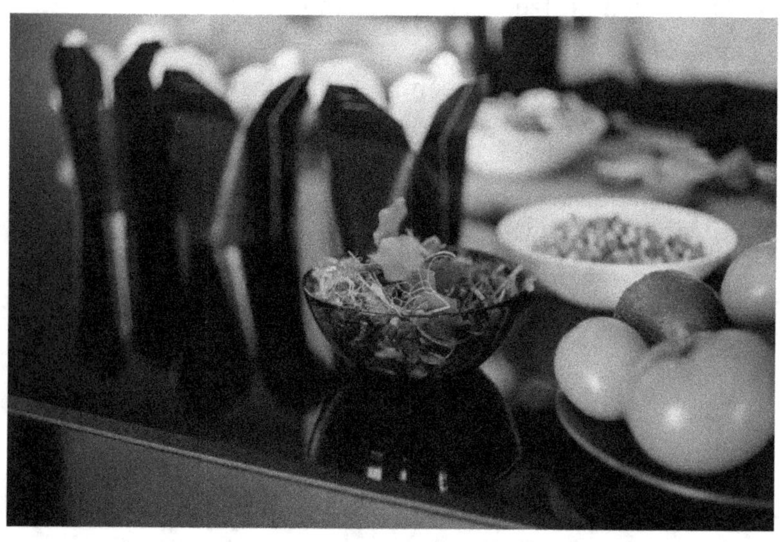

CHAPTER 4

Safety and Considerations of Intermittent Fasting

If you're considering intermittent fasting as a lifestyle, it's important to address safety concerns and understand who should approach this eating pattern with caution. While intermittent fasting is generally safe for most people, there are a few cases where it may not be suitable.

Who Should Approach Intermittent Fasting with Caution?

Children: Since children are in a crucial phase of growth and development, they require adequate calorie intake, essential nutrients, and sufficient protein. Restricting their eating window may interfere with their nutritional needs, potentially leading to health issues and growth problems.

While some experts suggest that children can safely fast, it should be approached with caution and under appropriate guidance.

Diabetics: Intermittent fasting can have benefits for individuals with diabetes, such as improved insulin and blood sugar levels. However, there are potential risks. Fasting may cause blood sugar levels to drop dangerously low, especially if medications are being taken to control diabetes. It's essential for diabetics to consult with a healthcare professional before attempting intermittent fasting and be vigilant about monitoring blood sugar levels and adjusting medication accordingly.

Pregnant and breastfeeding women: Nutrition plays a critical role during pregnancy and breastfeeding as the mother's body needs to support both herself and the developing baby. Intermittent fasting may make it challenging to meet the increased calorie and nutrient requirements during these periods.

Medical professionals typically recommend against intermittent fasting for pregnant and breastfeeding women to ensure sufficient nutrition for both mother and child.

Can Intermittent Fasting Trigger Eating Disorders?

While intermittent fasting works well for most individuals, those with a predisposition to disordered eating patterns should be cautious. For individuals prone to developing eating disorders, the focus on restriction and avoiding food during fasting periods can trigger anxiety, fatigue, mood swings, and disruptions in sleep and menstrual cycles.

It's crucial to be aware of any signs that intermittent fasting may be leading to disordered eating patterns and to seek appropriate support if needed.

Potential Side Effects of Intermittent Fasting

Intermittent fasting, like any dietary approach, can have side effects that vary among individuals. Some common side effects include:

Hunger-related mood changes: Feeling grumpy, irritable, or experiencing brain fog and fatigue due to hunger.

Low blood sugar symptoms: Dizziness, headaches, nausea, or fatigue caused by low blood sugar levels.

Obsession with food: Constantly thinking about what and how much you can eat during the eating window.

Nutrient deficiencies: Hair loss or other symptoms related to inadequate intake of essential nutrients.

Menstrual cycle changes: Rapid weight loss from intermittent fasting may lead to irregular menstrual cycles.

Digestive issues: Constipation can occur due to a lack of fiber, protein, vitamins, or inadequate fluid intake.

It's important to note that most people do not experience severe or long-lasting side effects, and these effects typically subside over time. However, if any side effects are severe or persist, it is advisable to discontinue intermittent fasting and seek medical advice.

Intermittent Fasting and Athletes

Intermittent fasting's effects on athletic performance are still under investigation, with mixed research findings. While some evidence suggests potential benefits such as increased growth hormone levels, improved metabolic flexibility, and reduced inflammation for post-exercise recovery, concerns exist regarding potential testosterone drops and challenges in consuming sufficient calories for muscle gain. Athletes should consider individual factors, consult with professionals, and closely monitor their performance and well-being when experimenting with intermittent fasting.

Is Intermittent Fasting Safe for Women?

Intermittent fasting is generally considered safe for women. However, some studies indicate that women may be more sensitive to signals of starvation, resulting in increased production of hunger hormones and potential mood swings.

Women may also experience hormonal imbalances and menstrual cycle difficulties with intermittent fasting, particularly if they have autoimmune conditions or pre-existing hormonal issues.

It is recommended for women to start with a gentler form of intermittent fasting, such as a 12-14 hour fasting window, and carefully observe how their bodies respond.

Remember, it's always wise to consult with a healthcare professional or registered dietitian before starting any new diet or eating pattern, especially if you have specific health concerns or conditions.

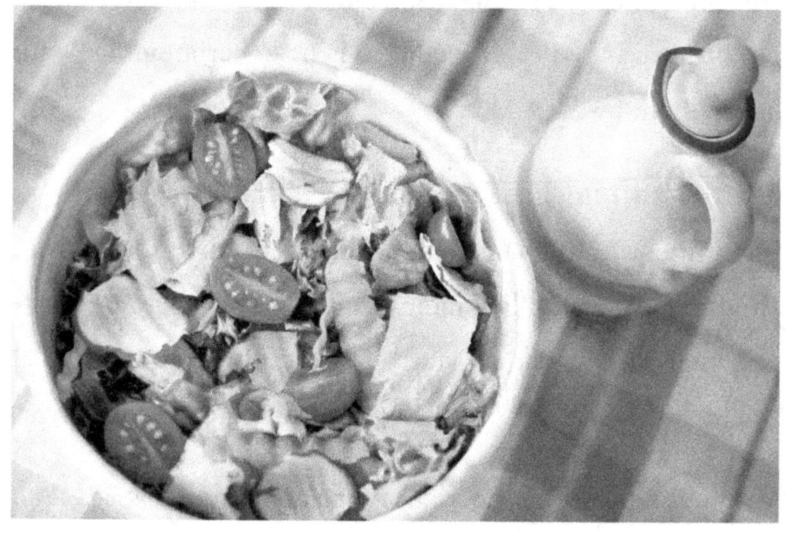

CHAPTER 5

Protocol for 16:8 Intermittent Fasting

If you're interested in trying intermittent fasting, the 16:8 method is a popular choice. This approach involves fasting for 16 hours and having an eating window of 8 hours. Here's a protocol to help you get started with 16:8 intermittent fasting.

Choosing Your Eating Window

When you're ready to begin 16:8 fasting, the first step is to choose an eating window that suits your preferences and lifestyle. This 8-hour period can be any time of the day. Consider the following options:

Noon to 8 p.m.: This allows you to fast overnight, skip breakfast, and have lunch and dinner at the usual times. You can even incorporate a couple of healthy snacks into your eating regime.

9 a.m. to 5 p.m.: If you prefer three meals a day, this window works well. You can have breakfast at 9 a.m., lunch at noon, and an early dinner at 4 p.m.

Afternoon to evening: Some people prefer breaking their fast in the early afternoon and having their last meal closer to bedtime.

Choose an eating window that aligns with your lifestyle and preferences to ensure you can stick to the fasting schedule effectively.

Planning Healthy Foods

To maximize the benefits of the 16:8 diet, focus on consuming healthy foods as much as possible. Prioritize nutrient-rich options to reduce hunger and cravings, which can help you sustain the fasting regimen long-term. Consider including the following in your meals:

• Fruits like bananas, apples, oranges, pears, peaches, and berries

• Vegetables like tomatoes, leafy greens, cucumbers, cauliflower, and broccoli

• Whole grains like oats, rice, quinoa, buckwheat, and barley

• Healthy fats like coconut oil, avocados, and olive oil

• Lean protein sources such as poultry, fish, seeds, nuts, eggs, and legumes

While occasional snacks and treats are acceptable, aim to balance your meals with a variety of whole foods. Minimize the consumption of junk food to avoid negating the benefits of the diet.

Choosing Calorie-Free Beverages

During your 8-hour eating window, you can enjoy your preferred beverages, but be mindful of their calorie content. To maintain the fasting state, consume only calorie-free beverages during the fasting window. Opt for:

• Water

• Green tea

• Unsweetened coffee

• Tea without milk

These choices can help control your appetite, keep you hydrated, and support your fasting goals until you break your fast.

A Sample Weekly Timetable

Here are three sample 16:8 eating timetables to suit different schedules:

Early Eating Meal Plan:

Mon	Tues	Wed	Thurs	Fri	Sat	Sun
8 a.m. breakfast	8 a.m. breakfast	8 a.m. breakfast	8 a.m. breakfast	8 a.m. breakfast	8 a.m. breakfast	8 a.m. breakfast
10 a.m. snack	10 a.m. snack	10 a.m. snack	10 a.m. snack	10 a.m. snack	10 a.m. snack	10 a.m. snack
12 noon -lunch	12 noon -lunch	12 noon -lunch	12 noon -lunch	12 noon -lunch	12 noon -lunch	12 noon –lunch
Evening beverages	Evening beverages	Evening beverages	Evening beverages	Evening beverages	Evening beverages	Evening beverages

Average Eating Meal Plan:

Mon	Tues	Wed	Thurs	Fri	Sat	Sun
9 a.m. beverage	9 a.m. beverage	9 a.m. beverage	9 a.m. beverage	9 a.m. beverage	9 a.m. beverage	9a.m. beverage
11 a.m. breakfast	11 a.m. breakfast	11 a.m. breakfast	11 a.m. breakfast	11 a.m. breakfast	11 a.m. breakfast	11 a.m. breakfast
2 p.m. lunch	2 p.m. lunch	2 p.m. lunch	2 p.m. lunch	2 p.m. lunch	2 p.m. lunch	2p.m. lunch
4 p.m. snack	4 p.m. snack	4 p.m. snack	4 p.m. snack	4 p.m. snack	4 p.m. snack	4 p.m. snack
6 p.m. dinner	6 p.m. dinner	6 p.m. dinner	6 p.m. dinner	6 p.m. dinner	6 p.m. dinner	6 p.m. dinner

Late Eating Meal Plan:

Mon	Tues	Wed	Thurs	Fri	Sat	Sun
11 a.m. calorie free beverage	11 a.m. calorie free beverage	11 a.m. calorie free beverage	11 a.m. calorie free beverage	11 a.m. calorie free beverage	11 a.m. calorie free beverage	11 a.m. calorie free beverage
1 p.m. snack	1 p.m. snack	1 p.m. snack	1 p.m. snack	1 p.m. snack	1 p.m. snack	1 p.m. snack
4 p.m. lunch	4 p.m. lunch	4 p.m. lunch	4 p.m. lunch	4 p.m. lunch	4 p.m. lunch	4 p.m. lunch
6 p.m. snack	6 p.m. snack	6 p.m. snack	6 p.m. snack	6 p.m. snack	6 p.m. snack	6 p.m. snack
9 p.m. dinner	9 p.m. dinner	9 p.m. dinner	9 p.m. dinner	9 p.m. dinner	9 p.m. dinner	9 p.m. dinner

These sample timetables can be adjusted according to your chosen eating window and personal preferences.

Remember, it's crucial to consult with a healthcare professional or registered dietitian before starting any new diet or fasting regimen, especially if you have underlying health conditions or concerns.

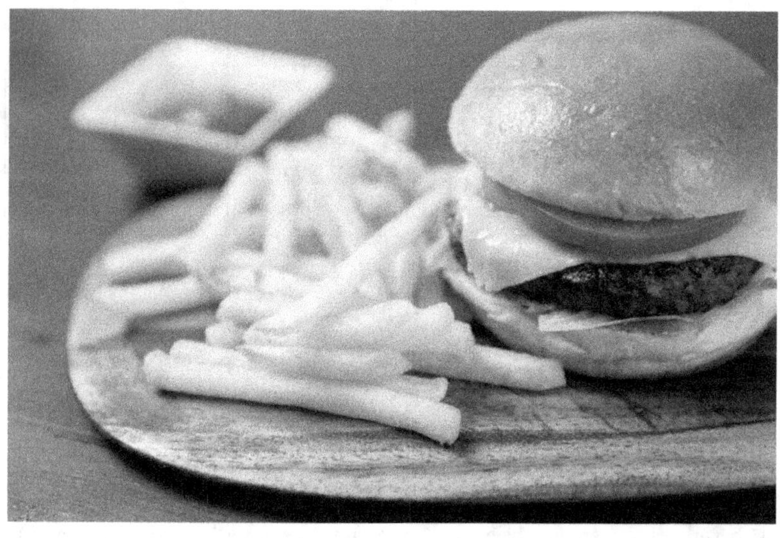

CHAPTER 6

A Protocol for 24-Hour Intermittent Fasting

If the 16:8 diet isn't suitable for you, you might consider trying 24-hour intermittent fasting, also known as the Eat-Stop-Eat method. This approach involves fasting for one or two non-consecutive days every week.

Introduction to the Eat-Stop-Eat Method

The Eat-Stop-Eat method was developed by Brad Pilon, who wrote a book about this way of eating. It is based on Canadian research into the effects of short-term fasting on metabolic health. The idea behind this method is to challenge conventional beliefs about meal timing and frequency.

Implementing the Eat-Stop-Eat Method

This diet is relatively straightforward to follow. You select one or two non-consecutive days of the week during which you will fast for 24 hours. On the other five or six days, you can eat normally, although it's advisable to focus on healthy eating for optimal results.

Despite the name, you will still eat on every calendar day when following this fasting method. Here's how it works: Let's say you decide to fast from 9 a.m. on Monday until 9 a.m. on Tuesday. You would have your last meal before 9 a.m. on Monday and break your fast with your next meal after 9 a.m. on Tuesday.

Staying Hydrated During Fasting Hours

During your fasting hours, it's essential to stay well-hydrated. Drink plenty of water and other beverages that contain no calories, such as unsweetened tea or coffee without milk.

Choosing Your Fasting Days

When practicing the Eat-Stop-Eat method, you'll need to select the fasting days that work best for you. This will depend on your personal preferences and schedule. Here are some considerations:

One or two days: Start with one fasting day per week and gradually increase it to two if desired. Avoid exceeding two fasting days per week.

Non-consecutive days: If you choose to fast for two days, make sure they are not consecutive. Extending the fasting period for too long can be challenging for most individuals.

Weekday vs. weekend: Decide whether you prefer fasting on workdays or weekends. Some people find it easier to fast during the weekend when they have fewer work-related distractions, while others prefer fasting on workdays to keep themselves occupied.

Experimentation: You may need to experiment with different patterns to find the fasting days that suit you best. You can try evenly spacing out your two fasting days or keeping them a day apart.

A Weekly Timetable

Here are some sample timetables to help you plan your 24-hour fasts:

One-Day Fast Meal Plan:

Monday: Eat normally from 9 a.m. to 9 a.m. (next day)

Tuesday: Fast from 9 a.m. to 9 a.m. (next day)

Wednesday: Eat normally from 9 a.m. to 9 a.m. (next day)

Thursday: Eat normally from 9 a.m. to 9 a.m. (next day)

Friday: Eat normally from 9 a.m. to 9 a.m. (next day)

Saturday: Eat normally from 9 a.m. to 9 a.m. (next day)

Sunday: Eat normally from 9 a.m. to 9 a.m. (next day)

Two-Day Fast Meal Plan:

Monday: Eat normally from 9 a.m. to 9 a.m. (next day)

Tuesday: Fast from 9 a.m. to 9 a.m. (next day)

Wednesday: Eat normally from 9 a.m. to 9 a.m. (next day)

Thursday: Fast from 9 a.m. to 9 a.m. (next day)

Friday: Eat normally from 9 a.m. to 9 a.m. (next day)

Saturday: Eat normally from 9 a.m. to 9 a.m. (next day)

Sunday: Eat normally from 9 a.m. to 9 a.m. (next day)

Note: You can adjust the fasting period according to your preferred timing, such as fasting from 7 a.m. to 7 a.m., 12 noon to 12 noon, or any other suitable hours.

Remember to choose fasting days and times that align with your individual needs and preferences.

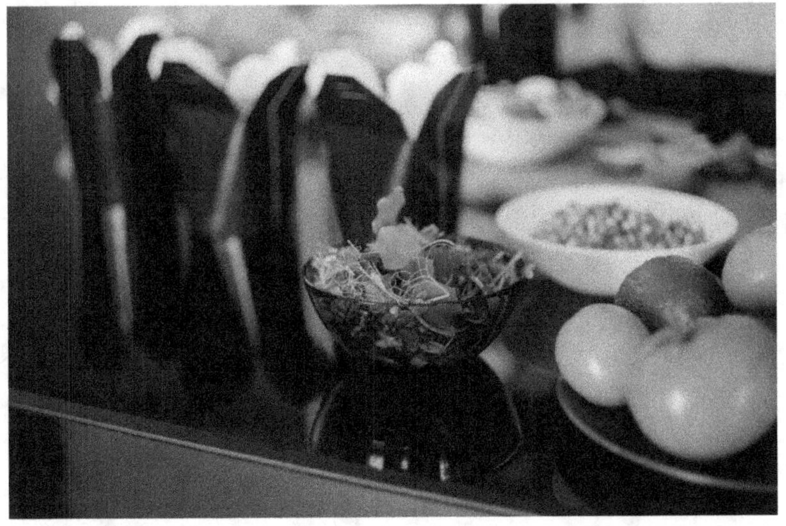

CHAPTER 7

Other Types of Intermittent Fasting

Although 24-hour and 16:8 intermittent fasting are the two most popular types, there are several others. Here, we'll take a closer look at five other kinds of fasting regimes that several people follow.

20:4 Fasting

20:4 fasting is sometimes called the Warrior Diet. It was one of the earliest diets to involve intermittent fasting. Made popular by Ori Hofmekler, a fitness expert, this diet involves eating one large meal in the evening. This large meal takes place in a four- hour eating window.

During the other 20 hours of the day, only small amounts of raw vegetables and fruits can be eaten. The food choices for this diet should be healthy – similar to those on the Paleo diet. They should be unprocessed wholefoods that contain no artificial ingredients.

A timetable for this diet looks like this:

Mon	Tues	Wed	Thurs	Fri	Sat	Sun
Midnight –4 p.m. vegetables	Midnight –4 p.m. vegetables	Midnight –4 p.m. vegetables	Midnight –4 p.m. vegetables	Midnight –4 p.m. vegetables	Midnight –4 p.m. vegetables	Midnight –4 p.m. vegetables
4 p.m.- 8 p.m. Large Meal	4 p.m. - 8 p.m. Large Meal	4 p.m. - 8 p.m. Large Meal	4 p.m. - 8 p.m. Large Meal	4 p.m. - 8 p.m. Large Meal	4 p.m. - 8 p.m. Large Meal	4 p.m. - 8 p.m. Large Meal
8 p.m - midnight - fast	8 p.m - midnight – fast	8 p.m - midnight – fast	8 p.m - midnight – fast	8 p.m - midnight – fast	8 p.m - midnight – fast	8 p.m - midnight – fast

5:2 Fasting

This popular form of intermittent fasting involves eating normally for five days every week. The remaining two days, calories should be restricted to 500 – 600. Sometimes called the Fast Diet, this way of eating was made popular by Michael Mosley, a journalist. Women are recommended to eat 500 calories on their fasting days. Men can have 600 calories on their fast days.

You can choose which two days you prefer to fast. However, it's best if they aren't consecutive. On those days, you can choose to eat one meal or two small meals. Many people prefer to eat two meals of 250/300 calories each.

This is a sample timetable for this way of eating:

Mon	Tues	Weds	Thurs	Fri	Sat	Sun
Eat nor mall y	Eat 500/600 calories	Eat nor mall y	Eat nor mall y	Eat 500/600 calories	Eat nor mall y	Eat nor mall y

36-Hour Fasting

The 36-hour fast plan means you'll be fasting for a full day. Unlike the Eat-Stop-Eat method, you won't be eating something every calendar day.

If, for example, you finish dinner at 7 p.m. on day one, you skip all your meals on day two. You won't eat your next meal until day 3 at 7 a.m. This equals a 36-hour fast.

There is some evidence to suggest this kind of fasting period can produce a quicker result. It may also be beneficial for diabetics. It may also be more problematic though since you'll be going for extended periods without food.

A timetable for this eating plan looks like this:

Mon	Tues	Weds	Thurs	Fri	Sat	Sun
Midnight - 7 a.m. Eat norm ally	Midnight -7a.m. Fast	Midnight – 7 a.m. Fast	Midnight - 7 a.m. Eat norm ally	Midnight - 7 a.m. Eat norm ally	Midnight - 7 a.m. Eat norm ally	Midnight - 7 a.m. Eat norm ally
7 a.m. – 7 p.m. Eat norm ally	7 a.m. – 7 p.m. Fast	7 a.m. – 7 p.m. Eat norm ally	7 a.m. – 7 p.m. Eat norm ally	7 a.m. – 7 p.m. Eat norm ally	7 a.m. – 7 p.m. Eat norm ally	7 a.m. – 7 p.m. Eat norm ally
7 p.m. Fast	7 p.m. Fast	7 p.m. Eat norm ally	7 p.m. Eat norm ally	7 p.m. Eat norm ally	7 p.m. Eat norm ally	7 p m Eat norm ally

Alternate Day Fasting

This way of fasting means that you fast for a full 24 hours every alternate day. Some versions of this IF diet allow you to eat up to 500 calories on a fast day. Others only allow you to have calorie- free beverages.

This isn't the best option for any newcomers to intermittent fasting. You go to bed feeling hungry several nights each week. This is hard to maintain in the long-term.

A timetable for this way of eating looks like this:

Mon	Tues	Weds	Thurs	Fri	Sat	Sun
midnight-midnight Eat norm ally	Midnight-midnight Fast	Midnight-midnight Eat Norm ally	Midnight-midnight Fast	Midnight-Midnight Eat norm ally	Midnight-Midnight Fast	Midnight-midnight Eat norm ally

Extended Fasts

Following the 16:8 or Eat-Stop-Eat method is quite simple. Some people, though, are keen to push the benefits of intermittent fasting to the limit. They prefer to do a 42-hour fast.

This involves eating dinner on day 1, say at 6 p.m. All meals would be skipped on the next day. On day 3, you would then eat your breakfast at noon. This would be a total fasting time of 42 hours.

If you try this way of eating, you shouldn't restrict your calorie intake during your eating window.

It's technically possible to extend fasts for longer periods of time. In fact, the world record stands at 382 days. Of course, that isn't recommended!

Some people do try 7 to 14 day fasts due to the theoretical benefits they are said to provide. Some people say that a seven- day fast can help prevent cancer. Others say that longer fasts promote mental clarity. These benefits are unproven and are theoretical. It's probably best, therefore, to stick to one of the tried and tested IF plans outlined above.

CHAPTER 8

Tips for Successful Intermittent Fasting

Now that we have explored different types of intermittent fasting, let's discuss some general tips that can help you succeed in your fasting journey, regardless of the fasting method you choose.

Start gradually: If you are new to intermittent fasting, it's advisable to start slowly and gradually increase the duration of your fasting periods. Begin with shorter fasting windows and then progress to longer ones as your body adjusts.

Stay hydrated: During your fasting hours, it's crucial to stay hydrated. Drink an adequate amount of water throughout the day to avoid dehydration. You can also consume calorie-free beverages like unsweetened tea or black coffee.

Eat balanced meals: When you break your fast, focus on consuming balanced and nutritious meals. Include a variety of whole foods such as lean proteins, fruits, vegetables, whole grains, and healthy fats. This will ensure that your body receives essential nutrients during your eating windows.

Listen to your body: Pay attention to your body's hunger and fullness cues. It's normal to experience hunger during fasting periods, but if you feel excessively weak or unwell, it may be a sign that you need to adjust your fasting schedule or consult a healthcare professional.

Be mindful of portion sizes: While intermittent fasting is not necessarily about calorie counting, it's still essential to be mindful of portion sizes when you break your fast. Overeating can lead to weight gain, even with intermittent fasting. Practice portion control and eat until you are comfortably satisfied.

Choose nutrient-dense foods: Opt for nutrient-dense foods that provide a wide range of vitamins, minerals, and antioxidants. These include fruits, vegetables, whole grains, lean proteins, and healthy fats. Prioritizing nutrient-dense foods will support your overall health and well-being.

Plan your meals and snacks: Plan your meals and snacks ahead of time to ensure that you have nutritious options available during your eating windows. This can help prevent impulsive and unhealthy food choices.

Manage stress and prioritize sleep: High levels of stress and poor sleep can negatively impact your fasting experience. Practice stress management techniques like meditation, exercise, or spending time on hobbies you enjoy. Aim for adequate sleep to support your overall health and well-being.

Stay consistent: Consistency is key when it comes to intermittent fasting. Stick to your chosen fasting schedule as much as possible to allow your body to adapt and reap the benefits of fasting. However, be flexible and make adjustments when necessary to accommodate social events or unexpected circumstances.

Listen to your body: Everyone's body is unique, and what works for one person may not work for another. Pay attention to how you feel during intermittent fasting and make adjustments as needed. If you have any underlying health conditions or concerns, consult with a healthcare professional before starting any fasting regimen.

Remember, intermittent fasting is a lifestyle approach, not a quick fix. It's important to find a fasting method that suits your individual needs, preferences, and goals. With consistency, patience, and a balanced approach to nutrition, intermittent fasting can be a sustainable and effective tool for improving overall health and well-being.

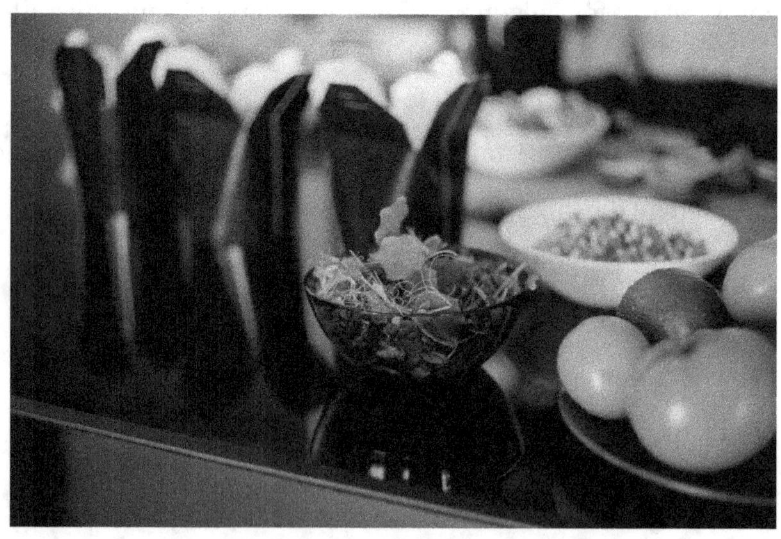

CHAPTER 9

How to Maximize Your Intermittent Fasting Results

Are you ready to try intermittent fasting? Whether you're doing it for weight loss or for other benefits, you'll probably want to maximize your results. Luckily, there are a few things you can do to get as much benefit as possible from your eating regime. Here, we take a look at some things you can try to speed up your weight loss.

Exercise and Intermittent Fasting

Research suggests that exercising while fasting can have additional benefits. It can impact your metabolism and muscle biochemistry, affecting insulin sensitivity and blood sugar levels. When you exercise while fasting, your glycogen (stored carbs) get depleted, leading to increased fat burning.

To optimize your results, consume protein after your workout to build and maintain muscle and promote better recovery. Additionally, follow up strength training with carbohydrates within 30 minutes of your workout. It's advisable to eat food close to any moderate or high-intensity exercise session and stay well-hydrated by drinking plenty of water. Maintaining electrolyte levels is important, and coconut water can be a useful option.

If you feel lightheaded or dizzy when working out while fasting, take a break and listen to your body. If you're doing a longer fast, consider engaging in gentle exercises like pilates, yoga, or walking, as they can help burn fat without causing discomfort.

Choosing the Right Regimen for You

To maximize the results of your intermittent fasting, it's essential to choose the right regimen that suits your lifestyle and makes it easier for you to adhere to the fasting schedule. With various types of intermittent fasting diets available, not all will be suitable for everyone. Here are some questions to help you choose wisely:

Are you already eating healthily? If you currently follow a standard American diet, which is high in carbs, sugars, and processed foods, it might be challenging to transition directly into extreme fasting. Consider starting with a shorter fasting window while detoxing from sugar and gradually incorporating whole foods into your diet. Once you've adjusted, you can increase the fasting window if desired. If you already eat healthily, you can start with a longer fasting window.

Can you manage to go for long periods without eating? Experiment with different fasting durations and pay attention to how fasting makes you feel. If extended fasts are challenging, consider methods like the 5:2 or 16:8. If fasting comes easily, you may be able to attempt a 36-hour fast from the beginning.

How does your schedule look? Fasting might be easier when you're busy and less focused on food. If possible, schedule your fasting period during work or while engaged in activities that distract you from feeling hungry. If you work out, you might prefer ending your fasting window immediately after exercising.

Considering these questions will help you choose a regimen that aligns with your life and preferences, increasing your chances of success.

Adding in Keto

Combining intermittent fasting with the keto diet is believed by some experts to enhance weight loss. The keto diet involves consuming most calories from healthy fats, a moderate amount from protein, and minimal carbohydrates. This low-carb, high-fat diet prompts the body to burn fat instead of sugars for energy.

When carbs are insufficient for daily activities, the liver breaks down fat, producing ketones that serve as an energy source. This metabolic state is known as ketosis, hence the name "keto."

Similar to intermittent fasting, the keto diet offers various benefits, including weight loss, improved blood sugar levels, and enhanced brain function. Many individuals claim it helps with conditions like diabetes and obesity.

By combining keto dieting with intermittent fasting, you can spend more time in ketosis, potentially increasing energy levels, reducing hunger, and accelerating weight loss.

Remember, it's important to consult a healthcare professional before making significant changes to your diet or exercise routine, especially if you have underlying health conditions or concerns. They can provide personalized guidance and ensure you approach intermittent fasting and the keto diet safely.

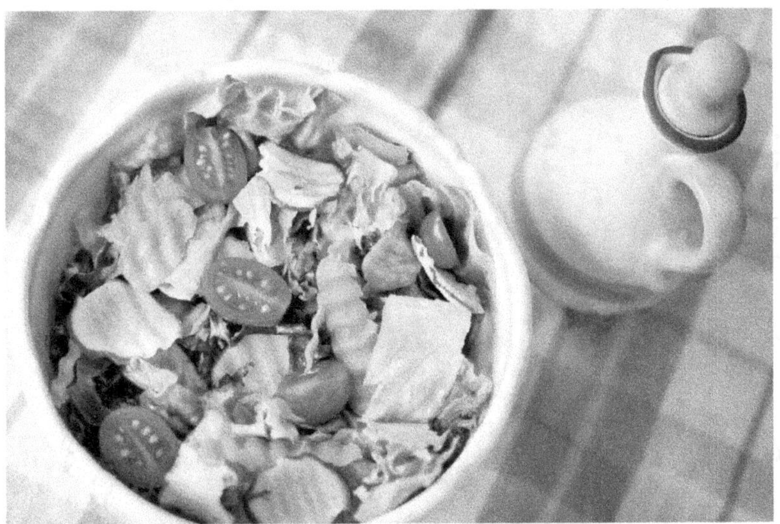

CHAPTER 10

How to get Started with Intermittent Fasting

If you're convinced of the benefits of intermittent fasting, you'll need to know how to get started. After all, embarking on any new regime can be complicated. So, how can you get yourself off to the best possible start? Here are some top tips.

Starting with a less Rigorous Regime

It may be tempting to try to lose as much weight as possible by starting out with a long fast. However, bear in mind this may not be the best approach. As we've already mentioned, it can be difficult to fast for extended periods if you've never done it before. If you're used to a high-carb, high-sugar, processed foods diet, you'll struggle to fast for 36 hours straight off.

If you find your first fast impossibly hard, you'll probably put off the whole idea. Even if you aren't, the likelihood of sticking to it for any length of time is low.

It's recommended to try any intermittent fasting plan for at least a month. This will give you enough time to see whether it's working for you or not. It will be very difficult for someone inexperienced to stick to an extended fast regime in the long- term.

It's therefore best to opt for one of the less rigorous regimes to start with. The 5:2 diet allows you to eat some food every day. In fact, you can eat your regular meals on five days of the week. The other two, you still get 500 or 600 calories to play with. This should give you plenty of options as long as you make healthy choices. Choose your meals wisely, and you'll experience the benefits without ever feeling hungry.

Alternatively, try the popular 16:8 method. For a large proportion of your fasting time you'll be asleep. You'll then be free to eat whatever you like (within reason) during your 8-hour eating window. Many people like the freedom that this offers. When they get used to the 16-hour fast, they find this way of eating quite simple.

If you want to work up to longer fasts once you're used to fasting, you can. However, many people continue to follow their initial plan in the long-term and experience good results.

Staying Hydrated

Whatever type of intermittent fasting plan you try, you need to stay well-hydrated. Fasting is only referring to food and calorie- containing beverages. It doesn't mean you can't have water and other calorie-free drinks. In fact, you should drink more of them!

Staying hydrated will ensure that toxins can be flushed effectively from your body. This will help to promote your weight loss and wellness goals. It will also help you to stay healthy in other ways. Your skin will be healthier. Your bowel habits will be more regular. You'll also avoid headaches and other problems associated with dehydration.

Drinking calorie-free beverages during your fasting window can also help to prevent you from feeling hungry. Often, we think we're hungry, but we're actually thirsty instead. If you drink a glass of water when you're beginning to feel hungry, you'll continue fasting for longer.

Try Experimenting with Different Eating Patterns

We have suggested some eating plan timetables above, however that doesn't mean you need to stick to them. The days and times that we have suggested are just examples. They may not work for you. You need to choose the right days and eating patterns to fit your lifestyle, preferences and needs.

Perhaps you prefer to begin eating as soon as you get up and then have your last meal early. Or maybe breaking your fast in the early afternoon and having a last meal just before bed is best.

You may prefer to fast at the weekend so you don't need to worry about feeling tired at work. Or fasting on a weekday may be right for you so you have distractions.

There is no single perfect IF plan for everyone. That means you may need to do a little experimentation. Weigh up the pros and cons of all the regimes that we've suggested. Think about which one you're most drawn to and give it a try. It's best to try to give it a month to see how well it works for you.

If you're having problems, it's time to go back to the drawing board. Try a different intermittent fasting regime to see if that better suits your lifestyle. Or move your eating windows around a little to see if it becomes more manageable.

Don't be afraid to experiment – after all, experimentation could be the key to success.

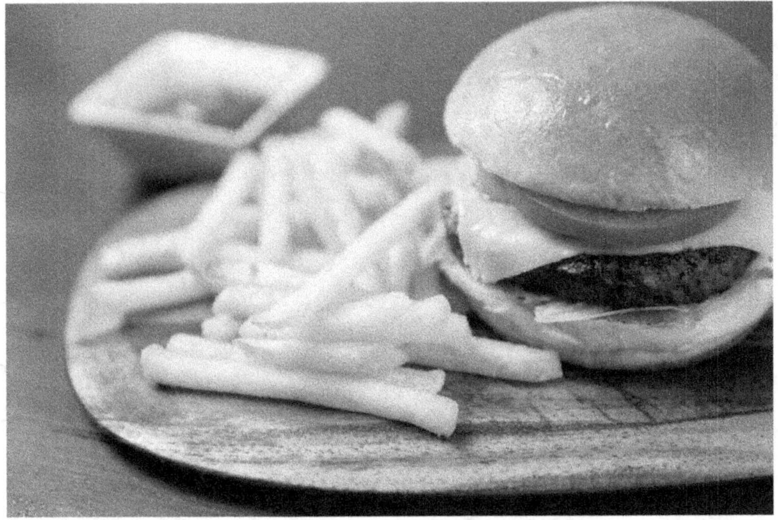

CHAPTER 11

Addressing Common Questions

When you're eager to start intermittent fasting, it's natural to have questions. In this chapter, we'll address some common concerns and provide answers to help you make an informed decision about whether intermittent fasting (IF) is right for you.

Exercise and Fasting

Many people wonder if they can continue exercising while fasting. In most cases, intermittent fasting won't prevent you from working out. It may take some time to adjust to your new routine, but some people even find they have increased energy while fasting.

Concerns about muscle loss during fasting can be mitigated by consuming sufficient protein during your eating window and engaging in regular resistance training. This combination can help preserve muscle mass.

It's generally recommended to exercise toward the end of your fasting period. You'll likely feel hungry about 30 minutes after your workout, so breaking your fast at that time can leave you feeling satisfied.

What to Eat During Your Eating Window

Intermittent fasting doesn't impose strict restrictions on what you can eat during your eating window. However, making healthy choices is still important to reap the benefits of IF.

A balanced diet with nutrient-dense foods is advisable. Opt for seeds, beans, nuts, whole grains, vegetables, fruits, and lean protein. Some foods that can be particularly beneficial when following an intermittent fasting lifestyle include:

Avocados: High in calories but packed with satiating monounsaturated fats.

Fish: Rich in protein, healthy fats, and vitamin D, which supports brain health.

Cruciferous vegetables: Cauliflower, Brussels sprouts, and broccoli are fiber-rich and can promote a feeling of fullness while aiding digestion.

Potatoes: Despite misconceptions, potatoes can be satisfying and keep you feeling full longer.

Legumes and beans: These low-calorie carbohydrate sources provide energy, protein, and fiber.

Probiotics: Foods like sauerkraut, kefir, and kombucha support gut health during the adjustment to the fasting diet.

Berries: Packed with nutrients, vitamin C, and flavonoids known to support weight loss.

Eggs: A quick and protein-rich option that promotes satiety.

Nuts: While high in calories, nuts contain polyunsaturated fats that help you feel full.

Whole grains: Despite being carbohydrates, whole grains are rich in protein and fiber, keeping you full for longer and potentially boosting metabolism.

Beverages During the Fasting Period

The beverages you consume during your fasting period depend on the fasting method you're following.

If you're doing the 5:2 diet, you can consume up to 500 or 600 calories on your fast days, focusing on low-calorie, nutrient-rich foods like vegetables and fruits.

For other fasting methods, solid foods and calorie-containing drinks are avoided. However, you can stay hydrated with various options:

Water: Still or sparkling water is suitable, and you can add a squeeze of lime or lemon for flavor. Be cautious with artificial sweeteners as they can disrupt fasting.

Black coffee: Contains no calories and doesn't affect insulin levels. You can add spices like cinnamon for flavor.

Tea: Oolong, black, green, and herbal teas are acceptable. They support cellular health, gut health, and probiotic balance.

Apple cider vinegar: Can be consumed to support blood sugar levels and digestion, potentially enhancing fasting results.

Bone broth or vegetable broth: Homemade broths without artificial additives can be consumed during longer fasts for additional nutrients and electrolytes.

Avoid calorie-containing beverages like "zero-calorie" sodas, coconut water, almond milk (due to sugar content), and alcohol, as they can break the fast and impact your progress.

Intermittent Fasting for Children

There is no specific evidence regarding the safety of intermittent fasting for children. Some experts suggest it may be acceptable for overweight children, while others caution against it due to their ongoing growth and nutritional needs. Consulting a doctor before introducing a child to IF is advisable to ensure adequate nutrient intake for growth and development.

Is Fasting Unhealthy?

Concerns about the healthiness of fasting are often raised, but fasting itself is not inherently unhealthy. People have been fasting for centuries without adverse effects, as observed during Ramadan studies.

However, fasting may not suit everyone's lifestyle, leading to inconsistent eating schedules and potential unhealthy consequences. Some individuals may struggle with recognizing hunger and fullness cues, which can be problematic in the long run and may lead to eating disorders.

It's important to exercise caution when approaching intermittent fasting if you have a history of disordered eating, as it can potentially exacerbate these issues.

Overall, IF can be beneficial for managing weight, improving metabolism and insulin resistance, reducing inflammation, and promoting cell repair and a healthier gastrointestinal tract.

Please note that before starting any significant dietary or lifestyle changes, it's advisable to consult a healthcare professional to ensure they are suitable for your specific circumstances.

CONCLUSION

By now, you have gained a comprehensive understanding of the benefits and potential challenges associated with intermittent fasting. If you feel ready to embark on this dietary approach, this book has provided you with all the necessary information to get started.

Before diving into intermittent fasting, it's important to identify your specific goals and reasons for trying it.

Whether you aim to lose weight, improve your overall health, or enhance focus and energy levels, having a clear understanding of your desired outcomes will enable you to tailor your approach and food choices accordingly.

As discussed throughout this book, there are various intermittent fasting plans to choose from. You should consider which plan aligns best with your preferences and lifestyle. Perhaps a daily approach, such as the 16:8 diet, suits your routine better. Alternatively, a weekly plan like alternate day fasting or the 5:2 method may be more fitting for you.

When selecting your eating window, take into account your daily schedule, hunger patterns, sleep patterns, and physical activity. It's crucial that your chosen intermittent fasting plan seamlessly integrates into your lifestyle.

If it feels too restrictive or difficult to follow, it may become unsustainable in the long run. Aim to stick with the diet for at least a month to evaluate its effectiveness for you.

Once you find the right balance, intermittent fasting should yield noticeable benefits relatively quickly. In addition to weight loss, you can expect increased energy levels, improved focus, and a range of health benefits.

These advantages encompass a reduced risk of developing diabetes, potentially extended lifespan, and overall enhanced well-being.

Now is the time to take action and give intermittent fasting a try for yourself. The benefits are waiting to be experienced firsthand. Remember, intermittent fasting should make your life easier, not harder. Embrace this new approach with enthusiasm, and you are bound to enjoy the rewards it brings!

www.ingramcontent.com/pod-product-compliance
Lightning Source LLC
Chambersburg PA
CBHW061457250726
48657CB00013B/1932